MW00928892

Gregory J. Bergel

Herbs for runny nose and cough

15 herbs
for upper respiratory problems

The information contained in the book is given to the knowledge of the author. The author excludes all liability for the application of the rules and uses of plants described in the book.

Photos: pixabay.com

jacek.marciniak@gmail.com

Contens

Treatment with herbs

Herbal medicine is a type of treatment that uses raw materials and plant preparations. It is the part of so-called natural medicine that is most scientifically documented. Treatment with herbs has a very long tradition, dating back to prehistoric times – as evidenced by the remnants of medicinal plants found in Stone Age sediments. Treatment with herbs was heavily criticized in the 19th century. In some countries it was even banned, it was believed that only official medicine, based on synthetic drugs, could be used for treatment.

In the late 1950s, the first scientific articles about the harmful side effects of synthetic drugs appeared. Adverse effects of these drugs, and even diseases associated with long-term use, have been increasingly identified and reported. This mainly concerned side effects such as damage to the liver, kidneys, or the haematopoietic system. Also, it has been noticed that in the treatment of chronic diseases the results of synthetic drugs have sometimes been poor, especially in the treatment of elderly people.

In this situation, based on new research methods, the use of herbal medicines was again started. It was also important that such drugs are cheaper than synthetic drugs, and in addition to active substances, they also contain vitamins and microelements. Plant medicines are also better absorbed by the body than synthetic drugs. A good example is vitamin C, found in plant materials such as rose hips. Its bioavailability is 3-4 times greater in the plant form than after the administration of the vitamin in a synthetic form. Herbal medicine comes in the form of two directions. The first is the traditional direction, the basis of which are solutions, infusions, decoctions. Medicines are made from single herbs as well as herbal mixtures. Natural remedies are popular because they are easy to prepare and have a long tradition. They contain many active substances, are usually mild and slow, and are often used in the treatment of chronic diseases. Herbal infusions and decoctions have a multidirectional effect, stimulating or equalizing the action of many systems. It is also important to stimulate the body's immune forces by providing many vitamins or minerals. The downside to traditional herbal treatments is that the treatment is long-lasting.

The second direction of herbal treatment is the production of modern forms of herbal medicines. This technology is based on the separation of pure substances with known physicochemical parameters and specific therapeutic properties. Such a drug can be accurately dosed, its effectiveness and interaction with other drugs can be tested. In the last few decades, many active compounds have been isolated from plants, several hundred of which are used for treatment. The most popular plant-derived medicinal substances are papaverine, morphine, codeine, cardiac glycosides, ephedrine, quinidine, ajmaline, vinamine, vincristine, and vinblastine. Some are produced synthetically like natural plant substances. Most medicinal herbs are harmless, but some herbs contain harmful alkaloids that can be toxic if administered incorrectly. Taking herbal medicines, especially those less popular, should be done after consulting a doctor.

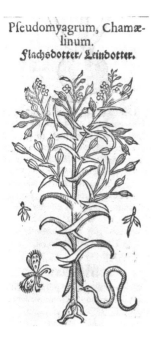

A drawing of a plant
in a 16th-century book

Eucalyptus

Eucalyptus (*Eucalyptus*) is a type of trees and shrubs. It comes originally from Australia, New Guinea and Indonesia. It is grown in Brazil and India. Eucalyptus oil is produced in eucalyptus leaves.

Eucalyptus is great for the respiratory system. Most often we can find it in syrups and lozenges, but you can also apply it as an oil on the skin (only in diluted form) to relieve inflammation and pain in the respiratory tract. Beware, doctors warn you never to take eucalyptus oil by mouth.

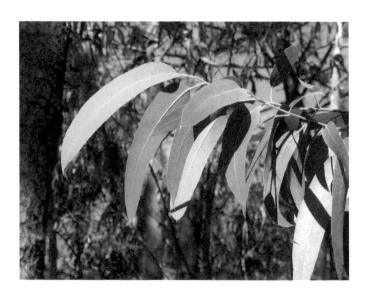

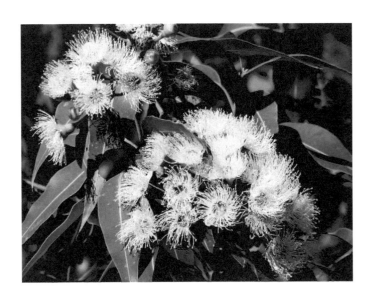

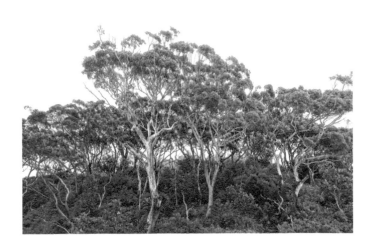

9

Lobelia

Lobelia (*Lobelia*) is a small, annual plant belonging to the Campanulaceae family. It is a group of over 400 species growing wild in North America, South America and Africa. It grows in wet meadows. It is often grown in gardens and balconies.

The plant forms dense clumps and carpets folded into slender stems. It grows up to approx. 20 cm. It has small, sometimes glossy leaves and blooms profusely. We can meet lobelia with flowers mostly purple and blue, but also white, pink and red. Lobelia can bloom from spring to fall.

Lobelia contains an alkaloid called lobeline which works to reduce congestion in the lungs and also re-

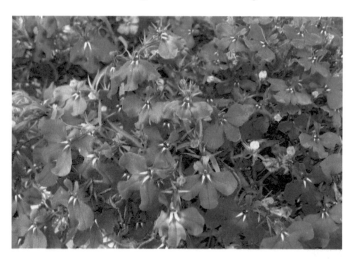

duce coughing by relaxing the muscles. Lobelia can be consumed in the form of tea, capsules, extract or tincture. Its dose should never exceed 20 mg. Ingestion of more than 500 mg can be fatal. Some species contain psychoactive chemicals.

Taking in the form of ready-made preparations.

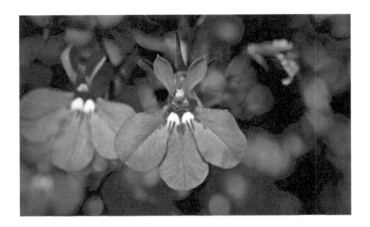

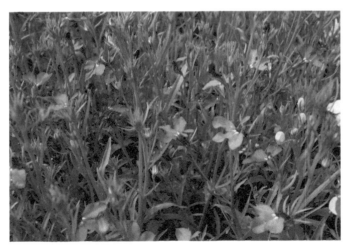

Oregano

Oregano (*Origanum vulgare*) is native to the subtropical parts of Eurasia. However, it is found all over Europe, northern regions of Russia and North America. It comes in many forms that differ in both plant habit and chemical composition.

The raw material is herb cut during flowering. It has a delicate aroma and a spicy, slightly bitter and burning taste. The active substances found in oregano stimulate the appetite, facilitate digestion and enhance the work of the intestines.

Marigold herb is one of the most popular spices in the world. It is primarily a characteristic spice of Italian cuisine, where it is added to soups, sauces, meat dishes and the famous Neapolitan pizza. Also

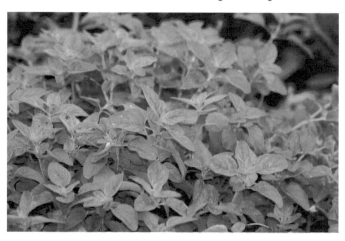

in Mexico, where some forms of the plant are still found wild, it is an everyday spice.

The action of oregano is very broad. It has antibacterial, antiviral and anti-inflammatory properties. Diluted oregano oil can be rubbed carefully into the chest or used for inhalation – it will open the bronchi or lungs and relieve the disease.

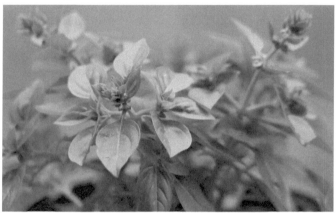

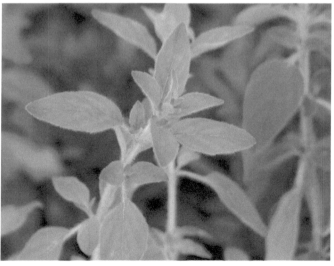

Spearmint

Spearmint (*Mentha*) – the genus Mentha belongs to the labial family. Within the genus Mentha there are a large number of species, both naturally growing and cultivated. Only in the temperate climate zone, 25 are known.

The most valuable is peppermint – Mentha piperita L., discovered in England in the 18th century and then introduced to cultivation on all continents.

This plant is characterized by dark green, strongly aromatic leaves. The leaves contain 1.5-3% of essential oil, the main ingredient of which is menthol. Menthol is a carrier of an intense fragrance.

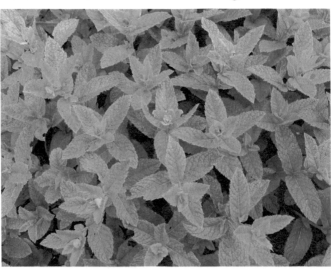

Mint is known primarily as a medicinal plant. It has a beneficial effect on digestive processes, increases bile secretion, improves appetite, and has a relaxing effect.

Menthol, which is in the leaves, clears the airways and makes breathing easier. It can be consumed in the form of: tea; oil that is rubbed into the chest (reduces congestion and soothes) and leaves.

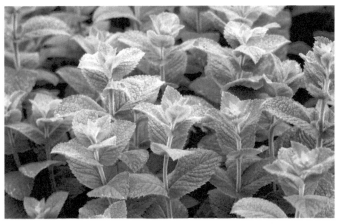

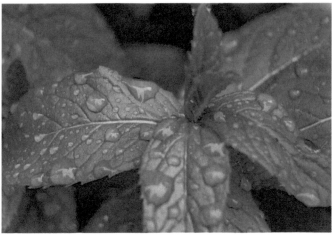

Plantain

Plantain lanceolate (*Plantago lanceolata*) is a common plant that grows in Europe as a weed. In the past, it was often used in traditional medicine to help heal wounds and relieve upper respiratory tract ailments.

It has an expectorant effect on the upper respiratory tract. The mucus substances contained in the plant cover the throat with a protective layer.

It improves the body's natural immunity by increasing the activity of immune cells. It improves the functioning of the liver and protects its tissues from damage. It has a beneficial effect on the gastrointes-

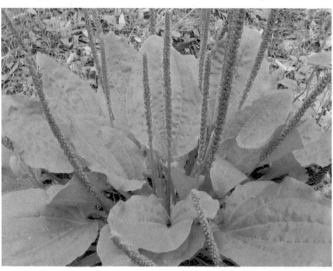

tinal mucosa and soothes gastric hyperacidity. It can be used in the case of gastric and duodenal ulcers. Applied in the form of compresses, it supports the healing of wounds, cuts and abrasions. It increases blood clotting and acts as an astringent on capillaries. It brings relief to tired eyes and soothes the effects of insect bites. Used for throat irritations, for heartburn and for the care of sensitive skin of intimate parts.

Plantain leaves contain aucubins, mucus and tannins that reduce diseases and infections of the upper respiratory tract. Tea from the leaves (dried or fresh) has antiviral and antibacterial properties, thanks to which it reduces inflammation and lung infections.

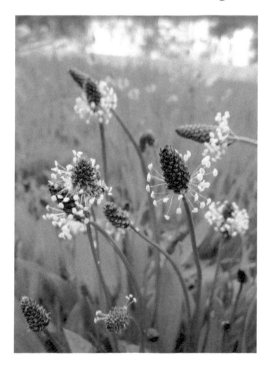

Osha root

Osha (*Linguisticum porterii*) comes from South America. It belongs to the celery family. It is 75-200 cm high. The ground part of the plant is similar to other celery plants such as dill, parsley or carrots. The root is dark brown, woody.

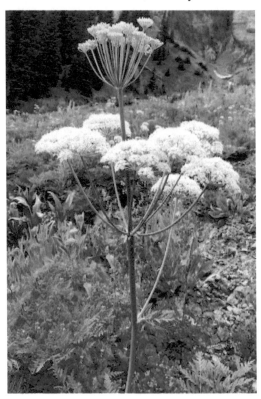

It was used in the medicine of the native people of America several hundred years ago. The Indians put osha roots and leaves at their newborn babies. They believed that the plant purifies the air these children breathed. Osha grows at high altitudes, above 2000 m above sea level.

Osha root is used for problems with the lungs and airways. It is used to fight respiratory infections thanks to its bacterial and antiviral properties. It has an expectorant and protective effect. Makes breathing easier. It is good for digestion. It helps to relieve cough, runny nose and sore throat.

It is used by people who practice mountain trekking – it facilitates breathing and prevents mountain sickness.

Osha root contains large amounts of camphor, which increases circulation in the lungs and reduces inflammation caused by allergies, asthma and pollen in the air. This root is most often found in lozenges and cough drops, which reduce the symptoms of colds and flu. Its anesthetic properties are especially helpful for a sore throat. This herb is also available in the form of tea, capsules and tinctures. Osha root should not be consumed by pregnant and lactating women.

Chaparral

Chaparral – evergreen plant formation, found in North America (western USA – California, northern Mexico), resembling a macaque. The plants that make up chaparral are high in essential oils and therefore flammable, resulting in numerous fires, especially in California during the dry season.

Chaparral herb is a medicinal desert plant that is native to Mexico and the southwestern United States. It is also known as creosote. Chaparral has an unpleasant odor and a very bitter taste, and the stem and leaves are covered with waxy resin; resin is extremely important for a plant's survival in the desert as it protects it from the sun's ultraviolet rays, reduces transpiration, and discourages animals from grazing on the leaves.

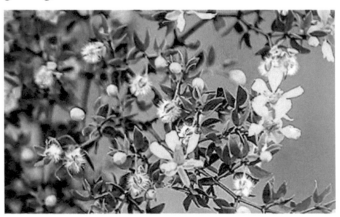

Chaparral contains a powerful antioxidant known as nordihydroguaiaretic acid (NGDA), and this chemical has strong antiseptic, antibacterial, and anti-inflammatory properties. Due to the presence of NGDA, there are many medicinal benefits of chaparral and it has been used since ancient times in a variety of medications. Southwestern American Indians regularly used chaparral herb for burns, skin eruptions, insect bites, and even snake bites. Other uses for chaparral have included applying resin from a heated branch to aching teeth and washing the hair with a resin solution to get rid of dandruff. Chaparral's hot herbal concoctions have also been drunk to treat colds, bronchitis, stomach aches, and diarrhea.

Czaparal contains NDGA and antioxidants that combat irritation of the upper respiratory tract and the reaction to histamines. This herb is most effective when consumed as a tea, but is also available as a tincture.

As further experiments proved inconclusive, chaparral was once again placed on the safe list, although caution is advised when using it.

Chaparral herbs should not be taken by very young children and people with kidney problems or lymphatic disease. While using chaparral, it is best to take it in small amounts. If you experience noticeable side effects, such as stomach upset, trouble urinating, diarrhea, and enlarged glands, it is recommended that you stop using the herb and consult your doctor.

Liquorice Root

Liquorice (*Glycyrrhiza glabra*) belongs to the Fabaceae family. There are many varieties of licorice, including: *G. uralensis*, *G. inflanta*, *G. glandulifera*, *G. typica*, *G. violacea*. Licorice is the most cultivated plant in the Mediterranean. Its natural area of occurrence is Libya, central and western part of Asia, Siberia, Mongolia, the Caucasus and eastern and southern parts of Europe. It is also grown in many regions of the world.

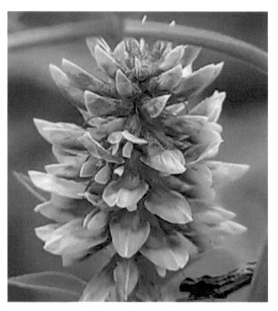

Licorice is a perennial that grows to a height of 1.5 m. The rather tall stem has alternate, odd-pinned, dark green leaves, consisting of 9-17 leaflets.

The herbal raw material is the root. Licorice has a strong expectorant, diuretic, antispasmodic, anti-inflammatory and anti-ulcer effect, protects the gastric and duodenal mucosa against injuries and infections. It stimulates the regeneration of the gastrointestinal epithelium.

Licorice is effective against: inflammation of the esophagus, stomach, duodenum and intestines, peptic ulcer disease, cough, spasms of the intestines, stomach, respiratory tract and bile ducts, hoarseness, runny nose, bronchitis, pneumonia, trachea and laryngitis, constipation, hyperkalemia.

This herb contains compounds that exhibit antiviral and antibacterial properties, thus combating the agents that cause lung infections. There are also saponins in licorice, which reduce congestion and bronchospasms. Consuming it as a tea soothes the throat and removes secretions from the lungs and digestive tract. It is also worth mentioning that licorice protects against the development of cancer cells in the lungs.

Contraindications: hypokalemia, hypernatremia, edema, hypertension, taking digitalis and diuretics causing potassium loss, renal and circulatory failure, pregnancy.

Thyme

Thyme (*Thymus vulgaris*) comes from the Mediterranean regions, grows in its natural state in Morocco, Greece, Turkey, Italy and Spain. It is cultivated in many regions of the world. This plant was already used in ancient Egypt, where it was used as a raw material for the production of perfumes, for embalming corpses, and also as a medicine.

The thyme herb harvested during flowering can be used fresh and after drying (it stays in the armpits for a long time). The smell and taste is strongly aromatic, slightly bitter. The raw material contains oil, the content of which varies within quite wide

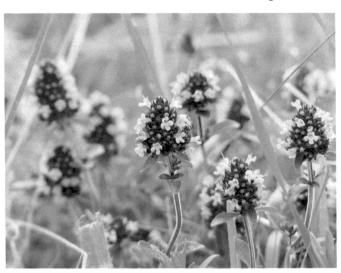

limits, from 0.75 to 6.3%, depending on the type of food, climate and harvest period. The main ingredients of the oil are: thymol and carvacrol, and there are also cineol, linalyl acetate, linalool and borneol.

Thyme has antibacterial, antihistamine, anti-inflammatory, antitussive and antifungal properties, making it a powerful weapon in the fight against colds, flu, sinusitis, asthma and allergic reactions. Thyme helps fight infections of the upper respiratory tract caused by viruses and bacteria, and removes residual secretions. It can be used in the form of an infusion, essential oil rubbed into the chest and an additive for inhalation. The leaves of the herb can be used to make tea. It is used for coughs, throat ailments, and to improve appetite and digestion. The substances contained in the leaves also have an antioxidant effect. Due to its properties, it is used to prepare a gargle, inhalation infusion, and also to prepare a hair rinse. Thyme should not be taken by pregnant women

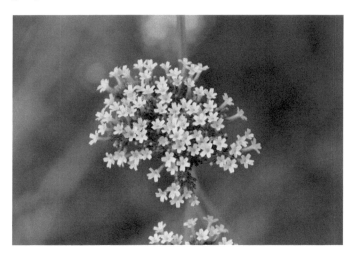

Lungwort

Lungwort (*Pulmonaria officinalis*) soothes irritations of the respiratory and gastrointestinal tract thanks to its high content of mucus. It is grown as an ornamental plant. In traditional medicine, the plant was popular as a remedy for coughs, hoarseness and other respiratory ailments. It was also used for stomach ulcers and to stop diarrhea. Herb infusions were used to wash wounds – astringent effect.

Lungwort contains a lot of mucous substances that coat the mucous membranes with a protective layer, moisturize them and soothe irritations present in them. It is effective in troublesome cough when the throat, larynx and trachea are irritated. In addi-

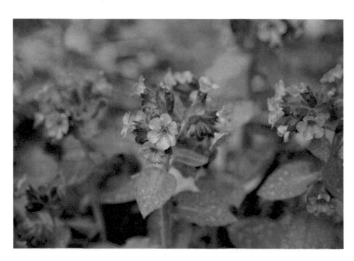

tion, mucus and saponins are expectorant, making it easier to get rid of the secretions in the lungs. Miodunka also has a coating and astringent effect on the mucous membranes of the digestive tract. Thanks to allantoin and flavonids, it improves the healing of irritations in the stomach and intestines. The tannins contained in the plant reduce the excessive work of the intestines. Generally, it is used to soothe coughs and hoarseness, irritated respiratory tract, irritations and cavities in the gastric and intestinal mucosa, and excessive intestinal perilosis.

Lungwort has strong antioxidant properties. It can be eaten raw, tincture or capsules. In turn, its leaves can be used to make tea, which will alleviate problems with the respiratory tract.

Preparation: 1-2 tablespoons of herb pour 1 cup of water, bring to a boil and cook for 10 minutes. Set aside for 30 minutes and strain. Consume 2 glasses a day in small portions (1/4 – 1/2 cup). Another way: cold extract – pour half a cup of herbs with 2 cups of boiled cool water. Set aside for 5-6 hours, strain. Drink half a glass twice a day. Can be refrigerated for 2-3 days.

Sage

Sage (*Salvia officinalis*) was a very popular medicinal herb in ancient civilizations such as: Rome, Greece, Egypt, India. In traditional medicine, it was treated as a cure for most diseases. It is known as a natural remedy used in the care of the mouth, gums and throat.

Sage preparations are used to rinse the mouth and throat due to its antiseptic and astringent properties. Sage helps maintain healthy mucous membranes, gums, and teeth. It has a good effect on the skin. It soothes skin irritations in intimate places.

Internally, sage alleviates excessive intestinal work and is beneficial for digestion and the functioning of the digestive system. It reduces the secretion of sweat and saliva. It also reduces excessive lactation.

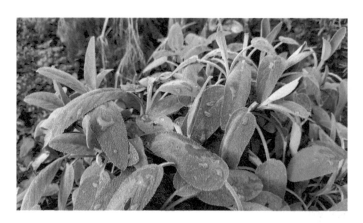

Sage also has antibacterial, antifungal, antispasmodic, anti-inflammatory, antiparasitic, antiviral, disinfecting, carminative and antispasmodic properties. Sage in the form of tea is the most effective way to treat breathing problems, sore throat and congestion. It is not recommended for pregnant women and nursing mothers.

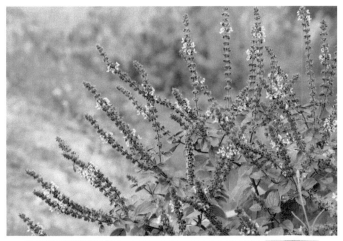

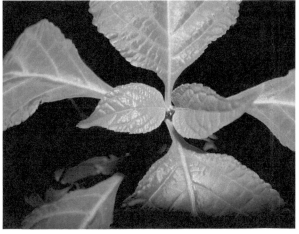

Great Mullein

Great mullein (*Verbascum thapsus*) supports expectoration, soothes cough, irritated throat, has an antiseptic effect. It was very popular in traditional medicine and in antiquity. In the past, it was also used for food poisoning and for liver ailments.

The mullein flowers are expectorant and help to remove secretions from the respiratory tract when you cough. They facilitate breathing, bring relief to a stuffy nose, soothe throat irritations. They are commonly used in herbal cough blends. Flower infusions are used to reduce immunity – they help the

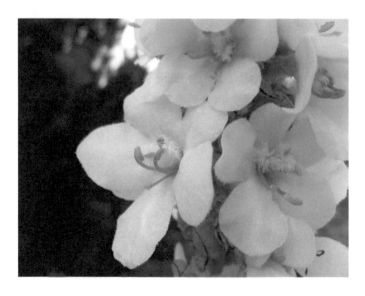

body fight viruses and bacteria. It has a calming effect.

Usage: pour 1 tablespoon of flowers with a glass of boiling water, cover, brew for 10-15 minutes. Honey and raspberry juice can be added. Drink 3 glasses a day in small portions.

Mullein leaves have similar properties. They can be added to or replace tobacco.

Mullein contains anti-inflammatory agents that cleanse the airways, strengthen the lungs and remove secretions from them. Mullein can be consumed as a tincture, but it turns out to be most effective in the form of tea.

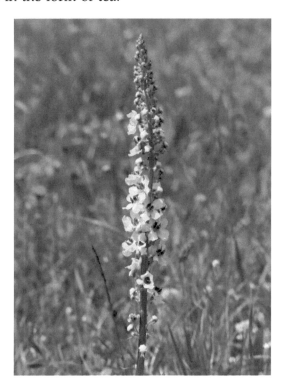

Elecampane

Elecampane (*Inula helenium*) was known in antiquity, used for medical and culinary purposes. The root was used during colds and flu due to its expectorant and diaphoretic effects. In the Middle Ages, Elecampane was added to wine to improve digestion and for its pleasant aroma. Elecampane is also used in Chinese and Ayurvedic medicine.

The saponins contained in the Elecampane root accelerate the removal of secretions from the lungs, and the essential oils stimulate the work of the snap epithelium of the respiratory tract and stimulate expectoration. The terpene compound (allantholactan) contained in the root has antibacterial properties.

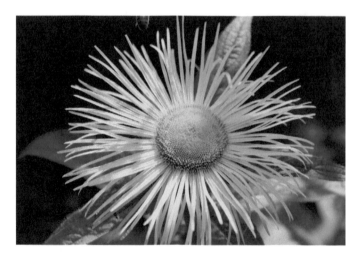

This compound strengthens the body's immunity and stimulates it to fight harmful parasites, fungi and bacteria.

Use. Infusion: 1 tablespoon of Elecampane root pour boiling water and leave, covered, for 20-30 minutes. Drink 3 times a day, the first dose on an empty stomach. Decoction: Boil 1-2 tablespoons of dried root in 2 cups of water and simmer for 10 minutes. Drink 1 glass 2-3 times a day.

You can also use leaves. For it to exhibit antibacterial properties that fight lung infections, boil the leaves and drink the infusion three times a day for up to three weeks. This herb thins and removes secretions and is especially effective in conditions such as bronchitis, asthma and severe cough.

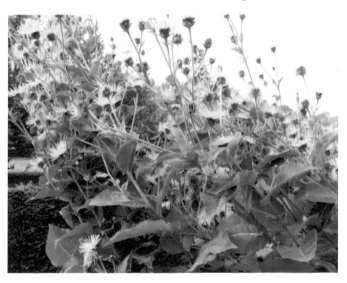

Coltsfoot

Coltsfoot (*Tussilago farfara*) has a positive effect on the respiratory tract. The ingredients of this plant contained in the leaves facilitate expectoration. In the past, coltsfoot was eaten as a salad in early spring. It was also used for lung disease as a tobacco substitute. In traditional medicine, it has been used to treat coughs, colds, strep throat, laryngitis, sore throats, asthma and other respiratory diseases.

Coltsfoot leaves contain mucilage compounds, tannins, gallic acid, essential oil, flavonoids, poly-phenolic acids, bitter substances (tusilagine), inulin, carotenoids and mineral salts. They have a beneficial effect on the upper and lower respiratory tract. The

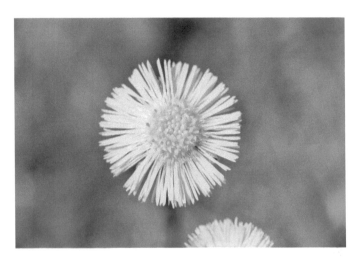

mucilages contained in it cover the oral cavity, throat, larynx and the walls of the respiratory tract, soothe their irritation and cough. They thin the secretion in the respiratory tract and support its expectoration by stimulating the work of the snap epithelium. Expectoration is also stimulated by coltsfoot flavonoids, which relax the respiratory tract and bronchi, making it easier to breathe.

The mucilages present in the leaves of coltsfoot protect the gastrointestinal tract. Their frequent consumption helps soothe irritation of the gastric and intestinal mucosa. Tannins have an astringent effect on the intestinal mucosa.

Coltsfoot leaves soothe skin irritations and facilitate the healing of wounds, corns and burns.

Do not exceed the recommended servings when used internally, because coltsfoot contains toxic alkaloids. Coltsfoot cannot be used for more than 6 weeks.

Use. Infusion: 2 tablespoons of dried leaves pour 2 cups of boiling water and leave to strain for 15 minutes. Drink 4 times a day in portions of half a glass. Honey can be added. Use a maximum of 2 tablespoons of dried leaves a day.

Cold extract: 2 tablespoons of coltsfoot pour a glass of cooled, boiled water. Cover and set aside for 6-8 hours. Drink 1-2 tablespoons every 3 hours.

It is not recommended during pregnancy and breastfeeding. If an allergic reaction occurs, stop the treatment.

Angelica sinensis

Dong quai – a species of plant from the Apiaceae family. It occurs naturally in China (provinces: Gansu, Hubei, Shaanxi, Sichuan, Junnan). It is a fragrant plant with a bunch of small white flowers. The flower belongs to the same botanical family as carrots and celery. Inhabitants of China, Korea and Japan dry the roots for medicinal purposes. It has been used as an herbal medicine for over 2,000 years. The medical raw material is the root.

Angelica sinensis is rarely used as a standalone herb. Most often it is included in various herbal mixtures. Therefore, some herbalists wonder if it really has a healing effect or only enhances the effects of

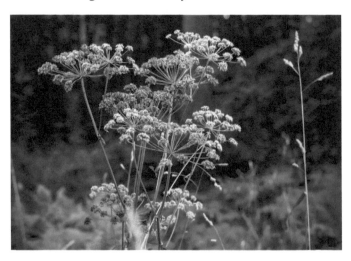

other herbs. Nevertheless, in traditional Chinese medicine, angelica is still used, especially in young women with menstrual disorders and in menopausal women, to alleviate the so-called outbreak symptoms, i.e. hot flashes, night sweats or mood swings. It is known that taking capsules regularly, drinking tinctures or herbal infusions also alleviates vaginal dryness during menopause.

This plant has an antispasmodic effect on the lung tissue and therefore relieves dry and sharp coughs. Thanks to its antibacterial and expectorant properties, it is the perfect solution for cloudy, transparent or white secretions.

Use. Tea: Pour 1-2 teaspoons of the root with a glass of boiling water and keep it covered for 20-30 minutes. Honey and cinnamon can be added. Drink 1 glass of infusion 2-3 times a day.

You can also eat the ground root powder – 1 g (about 1/4 flat teaspoon) 3 times a day.

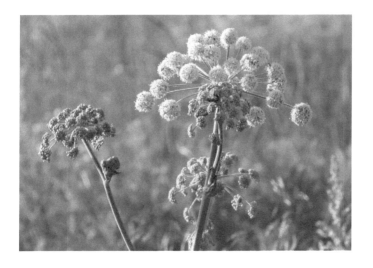

The following books have been published
in the Home Herbarium series:

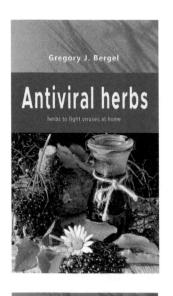

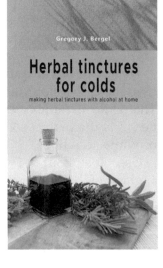

Short excerpts from these books will be presented on the following pages.

———————————➤

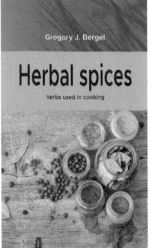

These books can be purchased on the Amazon platform – as paperback and Kindle.

Descriptions of herbs

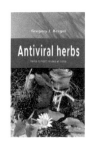

Aesculus hippocastanum L. – horse chestnut

Characteristic. The horse chestnut tree is a species of tree native to the Balkan Peninsula, where it grows wild and is at risk of extinction. In Europe, it was planted in parks and along roads from the 16th century. It is now common in urban areas, mainly in Europe and North America, as an ornamental tree. It is a tree up to 25 m high. It has a short and thick trunk, splitting into several thick branches. The bark is gray-brown, cracked. The crown is large, with dense foliage. Reaches the age of 200 years. Since the end of the 20th century, chestnut trees in Europe have been destroyed by the larvae of a small butterfly, which eat the leaves.

Herb raw material. The medicinal raw material of horse chestnut is: flowers, bark, seeds (the so-called chestnut), unripe chestnut fruit. The flowers are harvested by cutting entire inflorescences in May, then single flowers are torn off and dried. Unripe fruits are picked in July, ripe in September when they fall off. The fruits are comminuted and dried at ambient temperature, then drying at 60°C. The bark is obtained from smooth shoots that are 3-5 years old.

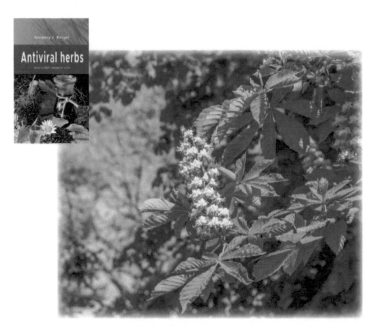

Medicinal ingredients. There is escin in horse chestnut seeds, which inhibits the action of hyaluronidase, which reduces swelling by sealing blood vessels, accelerates the absorption of hematomas, soothes inflammation of blood vessels, increases the tension and elasticity of the vein walls (and thus strengthens them), improves local blood flow, improves peripheral circulation, blood supply to the skin and smooth muscles. The mechanism of action is based on the inhibition of the action of hyaluronidase. It is an enzyme that deals with the degradation of proteoglycans that give stiffness and tension to blood vessel walls. Increased hyaluronidase activity is found in patients with varicose veins. The effectiveness of escin in alleviating clinical symptoms in patients with chronic venous insufficiency has been

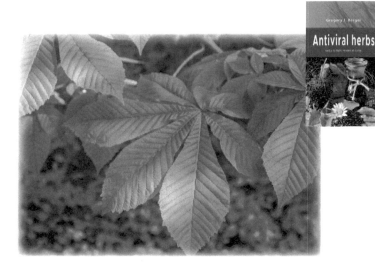

confirmed in randomized trials. Limb volume reduction, pain sensation and itching symptoms have been documented. Escin may enhance the effects of oral anticoagulants and the nephrotoxicity of aminoglycosides.

The bark preparations contain esculin and other coumarins and tannins, which have a stronger anti-exudative and anti-inflammatory effect than escin. Aesculin seals capillary blood vessels and has a strong protective effect against ultraviolet radiation.

The flowers are used in the form of infusions, they contain mainly flavonoids and improve the condition of the capillaries (reduce their permeability and brittleness).

Impact on the body, methods of preparation. Preparations with escin have been used since the nineteenth century for varicose veins of the lower ex-

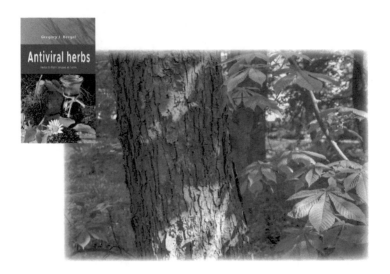

tremities and anus, inflammation of blood vessels, post-traumatic and postoperative conditions, edema of various origins and blood circulation disorders. Incidentally, it is used in brain disorders caused by various causes (stroke, trauma or inflammation), in brain edema, in pains caused by diseases of the spine. The daily therapeutic dose of escin is 15-30 mg.

Preparations from the bark with esculin are also used in the treatment of haemorrhoids, and in addition to inhibit minor bleeding, in gastrointestinal catarrh, diarrhea and ulceration of the large intestine.

Flower infusions compresses are used externally for abrasions, burns, frostbites, focal capillary inflammations and various contusions.

Chestnut flower tincture was used as an aphrodisiac. The tincture was also used externally with varicose veins in the form of compresses, and in infectious and rheumatic diseases.

It is believed that horse chestnut may be effective against viral infections caused by viruses such as SARS. It works by blocking viruses from joining the so-called 2 type of angiotensin converting enzyme ACE2 on the cell surface.

Contraindications and side effects. Chestnut preparations cannot be used by people with acute renal failure and by women in the first trimester of pregnancy (later and during feeding, they can only be used on the recommendation of a doctor). Chestnut preparations should not be used on damaged skin and wounds; contact of such drugs with the eyes and mucous membranes should be avoided. Some people may develop allergic reactions and digestive system disorders.

Herbal blends for hemorrhoids with horse chestnut flower:

A herbal mixture for sit-ons: yarrow herb, horse chestnut flower, oak bark, sage leaf, cinquefoil rhizome, knotweed herb. Pour a few tablespoons of herbs with approx. 2 liters of water, bring to a boil. The decoction is used for sit-ins. Repeat every day for 5 to 7 days.

A herbal mixture for washing: chamomile basket, chestnut flower, sage leaf. Pour one tablespoon of herbs into a glass of hot water. The decoction should be used for washes and compresses

Chestnut tincture improves blood flow, prevents swelling and varicose veins. It can be used for rubbing in the event of muscle and joint pain.
• Crush a dozen or so ripe chestnuts, pour a glass of boiled, cold water and ½ l of spirit.

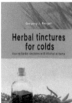

Rosehip tincture

Rosehip (*Rosa canina* L.) grows in temperate and warm areas of the Northern Hemisphere. It can be found almost all over Europe, North Africa, the Canary Islands, Madeira, Asia, Australia, and New Zealand. It is a shrub that often grows on the edge of forests and in roadside thickets. It has beautifully fragrant flowers in summer, and in autumn it has characteristic oblong red fruit. The fruit acquires its healing properties after being frozen. They are a great delicacy of birds, so it is better not to wait until the first frost to harvest. You can pick rosehips earlier and freeze them in your home freezer.

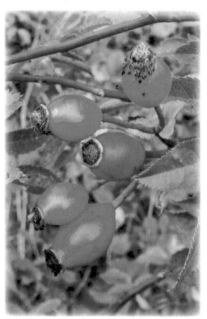

Tincture 1.

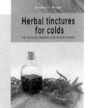

Ingredients:

2 pounds of rose hips,
3 cups of spirit 96%,
2 cups of vodka 40%,
2 cups of light honey,
2 cups of water,
5 cloves,
1 teaspoon of dried mint,
1 teaspoon of the dried chamomile flower.

Wash the rosehips, dry them, and put them in the freezer for a day. Puncture with a pin, add to the jar, add the herbs, pour the spirit over it. Keep warm for 4-6 weeks, shaking the jar every few days. Strain, squeezing the fruit juice, set aside for a week, and filter a few times. Mix honey with warm water, heat up, and collect scum. When it cools down, add vodka and combine with the previously prepared spirit with the rose. The tincture must mature in a cool place for at least 2 months.

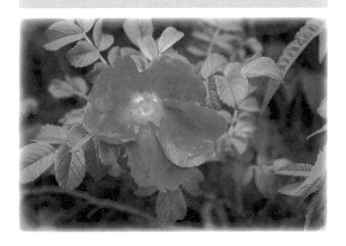

Tincture 2.

This tincture has a unique aroma due to its herbal content.

Ingredients:

2 pounds of rosehips,
3 cups of spirit,
2 cups of vodka,
2 cups of honey,
6 cloves,
1 teaspoon of dried chamomile flower,
1 teaspoon of mint.

Wash the rosehips and prick them with a pin. Pour into the jar with the mint, chamomile, and cloves, and pour over the spirit. Screw the jar on and set aside in a warm place for 5 weeks. After this time, decant the tincture. Squeeze the fruit, strain the juice obtained, and combine with the previously poured liquid. Mix the honey with two glasses of boiled water to make it thin, cool, add the vodka, and combine with the tincture. Mix everything, filter, then pour into bottles. You can eat it after spilling it, but it is better to wait for about a month – it will be tastier.

Tincture 3.

Ingredients:
2 pounds of rosehips,
2 ounces of sugar,
4 cups of wine or vodka.

Wash, drain and crush the rosehips. Transfer to a jar, add sugar. Pour a liter of wine or vodka. Set aside in a warm place for a week. Drain through cheesecloth. Drink 1 glass a day.

Description of spices

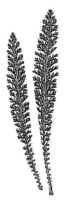

Herbal spices

Achillea millefolium L.

Common yarrow

A species from the *Asteraceae* family. It is common in Eurasia (to the east it reaches Mongolia and northwest India) and in North America (south to Guatemala). It occurs in pastures, meadows and wastelands from lowlands to mountain areas. Present as a weed on farmland. It grows mostly in areas with a suboceanic and moderately continental climate. Easily adapts to various conditions.

The seasoning is young leaves with a bitter, spicy flavor. Can be used as an addition to sauces and soups. It contains essential oils and bitter substances. It is added to herbal digestive and sedative preparations.

It is added to soothing and regenerating masks, creams and face lotions. It can also be a component of shampoos and toothpastes, and as one of many ingredients it is used to prepare relaxing baths.

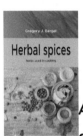
Acorus calamus L.

Calamus

Calamus belongs to the *Acoraceae* family. The species ranges from Asia and North America, and has been dragged and spread by humans to other continents from subtropical to temperate zones. It probably came to Europe between the Middle Ages and the 16th century. It is an edible, cosmetic and medicinal plant with wide applications in various cultures around the world.

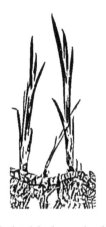

Calamus is a perennial with a thick, highly branched, creeping rhizome, up to 3 cm in diameter. It has a characteristic, aromatic, pleasant smell. Leaves are strongly elongated, 60-120 cm long and up to 2 cm wide, red at the base, otherwise light green. The bulb of the inflorescence sticks out from the axis of the shoot, green-yellow, 4-8 cm long; leaf-like scabbard.

One of the oldest mentions of the medicinal use of calamus comes from India, where the plant was used for healing in Ayurvedic medicine. This plant was also used in the ancient civilizations of the Mediterranean basin. It was found, for example, in the tomb of Tutankhamun. Calamus is a useful plant in various cultures, from American Indians to Chinese, Indians and Europeans. It was widely used as a medicinal and cosmetic plant. The rhizome is used to flavor sugars, tinctures and liqueurs. The raw material is obtained from crops (especially in the subtropical and tropical zones) or from the wild state (e.g. in Central Europe).

The plant – apart from its intense aroma and healing properties – also contains a toxin, so it should be used only in small amounts as a seasoning, not a main course. You eat the rhizomes, the young part of which can also be eaten raw. Calamus is recommended as an addition to drinks (e.g. compotes, liqueurs and teas), salads, cakes and puddings. Rhizomes were also used to make dry jam and candies (as a result of candying), they were also added to gin and beer. Calamus is relatively often used in Arab and Indian cuisines, where ground rhizomes are used to flavor sweets and fruit compotes. It is also included in herbal curry blends, mixed with nutmeg, vanilla and cinnamon. It was used as food by the Abenak and Dakota Indians. The Western Dakota (Lakota) group also ate leaves. In countries where it is allowed, powdered rhizome is sometimes a component of spice mixtures.

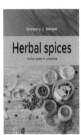

Alliaria petiolata (M. Bieb.) Cavara et Grande

Garlic mustard

A species from the *Brassicaceae* family. It occurs in Europe, North Africa, as well as in Western and Southern Asia. The invasive plant is found in the USA, Canada and Argentina as an imported species.

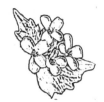

The aboveground part of the plant contains an oil with a very pungent taste, aliaroside flavonoid, and isosulfocyanine glycoside. Gluconasturcin was found in the roots and cardenolides in the seeds. When eaten by cows, it may cause the milk to taste unpleasant.

The leaves of the plant are used in France as an ingredient in salads. It is also used as a spice. Formerly used to pouch purulent and difficult to heal wounds and ulcers.

Hello!

Thanks for reading this book.

Since you made it to the end, I hope you found this book interesting.

I would like to ask you to leave your opinion on this book.

Why your opinion is important:

- it is an important signal to the author about the quality of his book;

- on Amazon, reviews are used to rank your book. It depends on whether the book is visible to customers or becomes invisible. A book without opinion becomes invisible to people browsing Amazon's resources. They become invisible just like unread books from "NeverEnding Story" or gods who no one believes in T. Pratchett's books.

Thanks to your opinions, the book is also available to other interested people.

Please leave your feedback!

Thanks a lot,

Author

NOTES

NOTES

NOTES

NOTES

NOTES

NOTES

NOTES

NOTES

NOTES

NOTES

NOTES

Made in United States
Troutdale, OR
07/27/2023